The 66 Change

Joshua Bassett

DEDICATION

In dedicating this book, I express my imperative to assisting others. My mission is to empower individuals through the application of my knowledge and experiences.

66

For 66 days

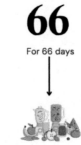

Eat quality food, no grains, no alcohol,
no soda and no processed
food(including sugar)

30 minutes of outdoor fasted
cardio and 1 high intensity
weights session in the evening

Drink an 0.5 oz per lb bodyweight
+ 12oz for every 30 min session

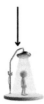

Do 1 or more methods of
biohacking provided

1 hour per day dedicated to learning
a new skill

Take 3 photos every morning
(your front, back and face)

CONTENTS

MEDICAL DISCLAIMER

The information provided in the "66 Change" book is for general informational purposes only and is not intended as a substitute for professional medical advice, diagnosis, or treatment. Always seek the advice of your physician or other qualified health provider with any questions you may have regarding a medical condition.

The 66 Change book involves suggestions related to lifestyle changes, biohacking techniques, and wellness practices. It is important to consult with a healthcare professional before starting any new health or fitness program, making dietary changes, or adopting lifestyle modifications. Individual results may vary, and the information presented is not a guarantee of specific outcomes.

The author of the "66 Change" book is NOT a medical professional, and the content is not intended to provide medical advice. However, the author is a fitness professional. If you have or suspect you may have a medical condition, promptly contact your healthcare provider. Never disregard professional medical advice or delay in seeking it because of something you have read in this book.

By engaging in the practices and recommendations outlined in the "66 Change" book, you acknowledge that you are doing so at your own risk. The author disclaims any liability or responsibility for any injury incurred as a result of the information provided in the book. Always prioritise your health and well-being, and consult with a qualified healthcare professional for personalised guidance if you do have health problems

PERSONAL NOTE

I'm Joshua Bassett, author of "The Metabolic Maze," and I'm excited to guide you through a transformative process that's all about reshaping your physical and mental well-being over the course of 66 days using 6 methods

In this narrative, our primary objective is crystal clear: to empower you with the knowledge and tools necessary for a comprehensive change. The focal point of this expedition is the synthesis of both physical and mental transformations, made possible through the adept application of six proven methods.

As we embark on this journey, each method is not just a theoretical construct but a practical roadmap. We're not just talking about fleeting changes; we're diving into strategies that will fundamentally alter your habits, mindset, and, consequently, your life.

My question to you is, are you ready to commit 66 days to a new and improved version of yourself? If so, let's delve into the practicalities, unravel the methods, and emerge on the other side with a revitalised body and a resilient mindset. The journey begins now.

1 NUTRITIONAL FOUNDATION

The first method of your transformative journey - a nutritional foundation rooted in quality fuel. In this method, we embark on a crucial exploration of how the food we consume becomes the bedrock of a profound metamorphosis. The idea is simple, which is focus on good, nutrient-packed food that's not just about filling you up but building a better you.

The importance of this method lies in a conscious and intentional approach to what goes into your body. We set a resolute focus on eliminating grains, alcohol, soda, processed and deep fried food from our diet. This isn't about imposing strict restrictions; rather, it's a purposeful choice to exclude substances that can hinder your path to transformation. Embracing a no-cheat regimen becomes the guiding principle, fostering discipline and dedication to the cause.

Why this emphasis on dietary choices you ask? Because what you feed your body has a direct correlation to how it functions and, consequently, how it transforms. By opting for nutrient-dense foods, you're not just consuming empty calories; you're providing your body with the essential vitamins, minerals, and macronutrients it craves for optimal performance.

Consider this nutritional approach as the architectural blueprint for your transformative journey. You're not just eating to stave off hunger; you're strategically fueling your body with the optimal nutrition it needs to thrive. This isn't a crash diet or a fleeting trend; it's a commitment to long-term well-being.

As you embark on this nutritional challenge, remember that this method is not about deprivation; it's about empowerment. You are taking control of your fuel source, aligning it with your goals, and setting the stage for a holistic transformation that extends beyond the superficial.

So, let's dive deep into the world of quality nutrition, where each bite is a conscious step towards a revitalised you. This method is not just about what you eat; it's about how you nourish your body, setting the stage for a transformative journey that begins at the very core – the food on your plate.

Grains, the seeds obtained from various plants, come in diverse forms, encompassing those with or without hull or fruit layers, all cultivated for human consumption. These essential food sources can be broadly categorised into four distinct classes: Cereal, oilseed, legumes and psuedocereal.

In 2002, a study suggested a connection between eating whole grains and a decreased risk of diabetes in men. However, the methodology raises eyebrows about the study's reliability. The researchers relied on participants filling out questionnaires every four years to recall their dietary choices over the previous 48 months. This method, based on intermittent self-reporting, introduces significant recall bias and potential inaccuracies. Relying on participants' memories for extended periods may compromise the study's validity, calling into question the robustness of the claimed association between whole grain consumption and reduced diabetes risk in men.

Grains contain prolamin proteins that bear a striking resemblance to opioids, triggering an increase in appetite and fostering a craving for more carbohydrates. This, in turn, often leads to overeating. Specifically, wheat houses gliadin, barley contains hordein, corn carries zein, rye possesses secalin, and oats harbor avenin – all types of prolamin proteins. Upon digestion, these proteins give rise to opioid-like molecules capable of binding to opioid receptors, intensifying the carb-craving impact associated with grains. This mechanism explains why the desire to indulge in dessert persists even after consuming a large pizza.

The objective here isn't to discourage carb consumption but rather to advocate for a shift away from grain-based carbs. Opting for fruits, whether sweet or non-sweet, provides a carb alternative that doesn't involve the prolamin-induced cravings associated with grains. So, it's not about ditching carbs; it's about making a carb-savvy choice that aligns with your health and well-being.

Over an extended period, excessive alcohol consumption can contribute to weight gain. Intensive drinking has the potential to trigger hormonal responses related to appetite, hunger, and stress. Additionally, alcohol is calorically dense but lacks essential nutrients necessary for overall well-being. In contrast, moderate alcohol consumption is not typically associated with weight gain. In such instances, the liver tends to prioritise metabolising alcohol over fat, hindering the body's ability to burn fat during drinking episodes. Furthermore, the simultaneous consumption of food while drinking is a common practice, contributing to the possibility of weight gain associated with alcohol intake.

I find it amusing when someone claims, "Processed food is good for you." My initial reaction is, "Is this person alright?" So, what exactly constitutes processed food?

To make a food product convenient to use, stable, tasty, and visually appealing, raw agricultural items are often subjected to various types of modifications, such as washing, cutting, cooking, canning, freezing, dehydrating, and packaging. Sometimes, different ingredients are added to enhance the flavour and texture of food products, often involving chemical processing. To maintain a standard quality-control protocol, almost all the food products undergo some degree of processing before coming to the supermarket.

Unprocessed food refers to food items in their natural state, devoid of significant alterations or artificial modifications. These include naturally occurring edibles from plant and animal sources, like fruits, vegetables, nuts, or untreated meat that hasn't been cured or subjected to preservatives or additives.

While I'm not here to judge anyone's choices, it raises questions when individuals consider products undergoing potentially harmful processes as beneficial. It's crucial to acknowledge the value of consuming unprocessed foods for their inherent nutritional benefits and the avoidance of artificial additives that may pose health risks.

It's essential to note that many processed foods commonly contain vegetable oils and linoleic acid. These ingredients play a significant role in various food products found on supermarket shelves.

The issue with this is that the surge in obesity is closely linked to the increased consumption of vegetable oil and linoleic acid, arguably more than any other dietary shift. This connection is noteworthy, especially considering evidence indicating that overall calorie intake, carbohydrates, sugar, saturated fat, and red meat consumption have remained relatively stable or even decreased in some instances, despite the simultaneous increase in obesity rates. Similarly, a substantial amount of deep-fried food often involves the use of vegetable oils and linoleic acid as well. These components are frequently employed in the preparation of deep-fried dishes, contributing to their flavourful but calorific nature.

Understanding the prevalence of these ingredients in deep-fried foods is crucial when considering dietary changes and their potential implications for health. The simplicity of reducing deep-fried food intake helps maintain a healthier balance, potentially benefiting cardiovascular health.

Imagine your body as a high-performance engine—a complex, finely tuned machine designed for optimal functionality. The fuel you choose to feed this engine directly influences its performance and longevity. Picture top-tier, premium fuel as nutrient-dense foods—meat proteins and fruits rich in vitamins and minerals. When you supply your body with these high-quality nutrients, it's akin to pouring premium fuel into the engine. The engine runs smoothly, efficiently converting fuel into energy, powering every aspect of its intricate machinery.

Contrast this with regular fuel, resembling processed and unhealthy foods—sugary snacks, deep-fried delights, and sugary beverages. When you introduce this type of fuel, it's akin to filling the engine with a lower-grade substance. The engine struggles to perform optimally; it might sputter, emit excess emissions, and, over time, incur wear and tear.

Now, consider toxic fuel—excessive alcohol, additives, and harmful substances. Pouring this into the engine is like subjecting it to corrosive materials. The engine's components deteriorate rapidly, leading to malfunctions, inefficiencies, and a shortened lifespan.

Just as a high-performance engine accumulates residue and damage from suboptimal fuel, our bodies accumulate the effects of poor dietary choices. Over time, the residue manifests as health issues, increased autoimmune conditions, decreased energy, increased rate of obesity, and impaired functioning of vital organs.

TEST YOUR KNOWLEDGE

Question	Options	Answer
1. What are the four classes of grains mentioned in the chapter?	A. Cereal, oilseed, legumes, pseudocereal B. Whole, refined, ancient, modern C. Rice, wheat, oats, barley	
2. Why is it important to focus on good, nutrient-packed food in the nutritional foundation method?	A. To save money B. To build a better you C. To follow a trend	
3. What is the significance of eliminating certain substances from the diet in this method?	A. Strict restrictions B. Enhanced transformation C. Short-term benefits	
4. How do nutrient-dense foods contribute to optimal performance?	A. They taste better B. They provide essential vitamins, minerals, and macronutrients C. They are low in calories	
5. What is the nutritional approach described as in the chapter?	A. A crash diet B. A fleeting trend C. A commitment to long-term well-being	
6. According to the chapter, what does the nutritional foundation method emphasise?	A. Deprivation B. Empowerment C. Indulgence	

Question	Options	Answer
7. Why is a conscious and intentional approach to dietary choices emphasised in the nutritional foundation method?	A. To impose strict restrictions B. To foster discipline and dedication C. To make the journey difficult	
8. How does the chapter describe the nutritional challenge?	A. Deprivation B. Empowerment C. A fleeting trend	
9. What does the chapter suggest about the importance of dietary choices in transformation?	A. They are irrelevant B. They have a direct correlation to transformation C. They hinder the path to transformation	
10. What is the guiding principle in the nutritional foundation method?	A. A crash diet B. A purposeful choice C. Indulgence	
11. According to the chapter, what is the emphasis on dietary choices about?	A. Deprivation B. Empowerment C. Indulgence	
12. How does the chapter characterise the nutritional foundation method's approach to transformation?	A. Difficult B. Easy C. Holistic	

Question	Options	Answer
13. What does the chapter suggest as a carb alternative that doesn't involve prolamin-induced cravings?	A. Whole grains B. Fruits C. Deep-fried foods	
14. What is the issue with excessive alcohol consumption mentioned in the chapter?	A. It helps with weight loss B. It triggers hormonal responses related to appetite C. It is not calorically dense	
15. How does the chapter describe the impact of processed foods on health?	A. Beneficial B. Neutral C. Potentially harmful	

Question	Options	Answer
16. What potential hormonal responses related to appetite can excessive alcohol consumption trigger, as mentioned in the chapter?	A. Decreased appetite B. Stable appetite C. Increased appetite	
17. How does the liver prioritize metabolizing alcohol over fat during drinking episodes, as stated in the chapter?	A. It doesn't B. It metabolizes fat first C. It metabolizes alcohol first	
18. What role do vegetable oils and linoleic acid play in many processed foods, as mentioned in the chapter?	A. They contribute to weight loss B. They are neutral C. They are linked to increased obesity rates	

ANSWERS

1. A
2. B
3. B
4. B
5. C
6. B
7. B
8. B
9. B
10.   B
11.   B
12.   C
13.   B
14.   B
15.   C
16.   C
17.   C
18.   C

2 DOUBLE THE BURN

In this section, we unlock the secrets to supercharging your fitness with a powerful combination: 30-60 minutes of outdoor fasted cardio in the morning and a high-intensity weights session in the evening. Understanding the science behind outdoor fasted cardio and evening weights isn't just about knowing what to do but comprehending why it works. Delve into the physiology of your body's response to morning cardio on an empty stomach and the impact of an evening weights session.

As you navigate through this method, envision not just a workout routine but a holistic approach to harnessing your physical potential. This isn't a mere exercise prescription; it's a strategic combination of movements designed to elicit maximum benefit.

The inclusion of this fitness duo in the 66-Day Challenge transcends the realm of physical transformation. It signifies a dedication to fostering resilience and a transformation in mindset. Over the next 66 days, you're not just checking off workouts; you're sculpting a lifestyle that prioritises your well-being. Each day presents an opportunity for refinement, for pushing boundaries, and for discovering the untapped reservoirs of strength within. My advice to you is, approach this journey not like a short test, but as a significant change that you feel in the rhythm of your heart.

Fasted cardio is a straightforward concept: it's about doing any form of cardiovascular exercise on any empty stomach. Typically done in the morning before breakfast, it involves a gap of 7-16 hours or more since the last meal or snack. The aim is to engage in exercise without recent food intake, prompting the body to use stored energy reserves. Whether it's a brisk walk, a jog, or a full-on cardio session, the idea is to break a sweat when your stomach is on the emptier side. The hype around this practice stems from claims that it may amp up fat burning and influence how your body handles calories.

Wait, Josh, I thought fasted cardio was just a myth? Well, let me break down the biology for you. When you go without food for an extended period, your circulating blood sugar drops, leading to a decline in glycogen (stored carbohydrates) levels. In such a situation, your body has no option but to lean more on fat, rather than glucose, to power your workouts, especially those lasting between 30 to 60 minutes.

 The science behind studies suggest that exercising in a fasted state encourages the body to tap into its fat reserves as a primary fuel source, potentially leading to greater fat oxidation compared to non-fasted workouts. This makes fasted cardio a better strategic approach for those aiming to prioritise fat loss and leverage their body's natural energy stores during physical activity. Overtime, concerns have risen, mostly often associated with engaging in fasted cardio is the potential occurrence of hypoglycemia, which refers to low blood sugar levels. Nevertheless, a majority of studies have indicated that participating in fasted cardio does not lead to harmful reductions in blood sugar, a reassuring finding even for individuals with diabetes.

 In fact, certain studies have gone a step further, revealing positive impacts on blood sugar regulation and insulin sensitivity resulting from exercising on an empty stomach. These findings suggest that fasted cardio might contribute to improved control over blood sugar levels and enhance the body's responsiveness to insulin. While these outcomes are promising, individuals with diabetes are advised to seek guidance from their healthcare provider before embarking on a fasted cardio routine. Consulting with a healthcare professional ensures that any potential risks or benefits are thoroughly assessed, allowing for a personalised and informed approach to incorporating fasted cardio into your fitness routine.

Well, when it comes to delving into the topic of fasted cardio, consider these five types of low steady-state cardio that seamlessly align with the principles of this fitness approach. Firstly, there's brisk walking and incline walking, a straightforward yet effective choice suitable for various fitness levels. If you prefer wheels, cycling, whether outdoors or on a stationary bike, is an excellent option to maintain a steady pace. For those who find enjoyment in the water, swimming offers a full-body workout with minimal impact on joints. Opting for an elliptical machine provides a smooth and joint-friendly exercise experience, ideal for individuals seeking a low-impact alternative. If the idea of easy home workouts is calling out to you, rope skipping proves to be an efficient and enjoyable way to elevate your heart rate. These five low steady-state cardio activities present diverse options tailored to individual preferences and fitness objectives.

Strength training proves to be a potent catalyst for optimal human ability, surpassing the impact of solely engaging in aerobic exercise. This heightened efficacy is attributed to the physiological effect of excess post-exercise oxygen consumption (EPOC), which remains elevated for an extended duration after strength training compared to aerobic workouts alone. The key lies in the fact that engaging in resistance or strengthening exercises sustains an active calorie-burning state in your metabolism for an extended period after the workout. Weight training is the secret key to unlocking a robust metabolic system. When you engage in weight training, you're essentially investing in building muscle mass. Unlike fat, muscle is metabolically active tissue, meaning it requires more energy (calories) to maintain. As you increase your muscle mass through weight training, your body becomes more efficient at burning calories at rest. This heightened metabolic rate becomes your metabolic currency, allowing you to expend more energy throughout the day and potentially supporting weight management goals. So, in essence, weight training becomes a powerful secret weapon in cultivating a metabolism that works for you.

Weight training not only acts as a metabolic currency for enhancing physical fitness but also plays a vital role in boosting immunity through the movement of lymph fluid throughout the body. The lymphatic system, a crucial component of the immune system, relies on muscular contractions to propel lymph fluid. Unlike the circulatory system, which has the heart to pump blood, the lymphatic system lacks a central pump and depends on movement of skeletal muscle, respiratory movement and smooth muscle contraction.

When engaging in weight training, the contractions and movements involved facilitate the circulation of lymph fluid. This, in turn, ensures the efficient transport of immune cells, nutrients, and waste products throughout the body. The enhanced circulation prompted by weight training supports the immune system by aiding the timely delivery of immune cells to areas where they are needed and facilitating the removal of toxins and waste.

Weight training stimulates the body's physiological responses, orchestrating a series of adaptations that result in increased muscle mass and strength. The process involves the recruitment of muscle fibres during resistance exercises. Initially, smaller, slow-twitch fibres are engaged for lighter loads, providing endurance. As the intensity rises, larger, fast-twitch fibres are recruited. Over time, the continuous challenge presented by weight training prompts hypertrophy, the enlargement of muscle fibres, as they adapt to handle heavier loads. Simultaneously, weight training triggers muscle protein synthesis, a fundamental mechanism for building new proteins within muscle cells. The mechanical stress and micro-damage incurred during weightlifting activate signalling pathways that promote protein synthesis. This process is vital for rebuilding muscle tissue, contributing significantly to both muscle growth and enhanced strength. Weight training also induces neuromuscular adaptations, refining the coordination between the nervous system and muscles. This heightened communication enhances the efficiency of muscle contractions and the recruitment of motor units, optimising force production. Due to the humans adaptive nature, we gradually develop the capacity to lift heavier weights, adhering to the principle of progressive overload—a foundational concept in fostering muscle hypertrophy and strength.

In the world of weight training, the focus extends beyond the traditional notions of heavy lifting and maximal loads. The key lies in lifting weights with strategic precision, emphasising time under tension, a full range of motion, and pushing muscles to the point of failure. This approach fosters not only strength but also endurance, sculpting a physique that reflects both power and resilience. My personal favourite method to training is a 4 second negative repetition, a 1-2 second hold followed by a 1-2 second positive rep.

Kettlebell training stands out as an effective tool for weight training. Their unique design allows for dynamic, fluid movements that engage multiple muscle groups simultaneously. Whether it's a kettlebell swing, Turkish get-up, or goblet squat, the emphasis is on controlled, deliberate motions that enhance time under tension and stress muscles across various planes of movement. However, if you are going to be swinging a weight that is too heavy with bad form, you may cause unnecessary stress on your spine.

While not traditional weights, bodyweight exercises form an amazing approach. Movements like push-ups, pull-ups, and dips allow individuals to control the resistance, ensuring that the muscles work through a full range of motion and experience prolonged tension. When I engage in bodyweight exercises, my recommended approach is to perform a specific amount of reps per minute, initiating the routine with a duration of 20 minutes and gradually progressing to 40 minutes.

Dumbbells are classic yet highly effective tools for this style of weight training. Exercises such as bicep curls, lateral raises, and tricep extensions can be performed with a focus on controlled movements. Adjusting the load allows for scalability and progression as strength and endurance improve.

Isometric holds involve holding a weight in a fixed position, maximising time under tension. Isometric holds can be applied to various exercises, such as holding a kettlebell in the bottom position of a squat or maintaining a static contraction during a dumbbell curl. These holds create a sustained challenge for the muscles involved.

Weight training extends its benefits beyond building muscles, positively influencing the mind as well. Engaging in regular weight training sessions has been associated with several mental health advantages. For those experiencing a low mood, engaging in weightlifting can be beneficial. A comprehensive analysis of 33 clinical trials, encompassing 1877 participants, determined that resistance training effectively alleviated depressive symptoms in adults. This study is under PMID:29800984. A closer examination revealed that these mental health advantages were particularly noticeable in individuals engaging in low-to-moderate intensity strength training. Moreover, those with mild-to-moderate depression appeared to derive the greatest benefits from such exercise.

When talking about the chemistry of the human body. As you lift those weights, your body releases a cascade of neurotransmitters and hormones, each playing a role in enhancing your mood and overall mental well-being. Endorphins, often referred to as "happy hormones," act as natural painkillers and mood elevators, providing a sense of euphoria. Dopamine, known as the "reward neurotransmitter," contributes to feelings of pleasure and reinforcement, creating a positive association with your workout. Serotonin, another neurotransmitter, promotes happiness and a sense of well-being. Additionally, norepinephrine, a hormone and neurotransmitter, plays a role in stress management, further supporting mood regulation. In essence, weightlifting becomes a holistic experience, not just for your muscles but for your mind, releasing a load of biochemical elements that uplift your physical and mental well-being.

THE FOLLOW WEIGHT TRAINING PROGRAMS ARE FOUND WITHIN THE JB ACADEMY.

2x per week

Given our limited training frequency of just two sessions per week, we've opted for a strategic approach to maximize efficiency and intensity in our workouts. Enter the realm of supersets, a method where we seamlessly combine two exercises back-to-back with minimal rest in between. This approach not only saves time but also ensures that each session is a mix of both strength and cardiovascular training.

upper body day

Superset 1	Sets x Reps	
Bench press	2 x 6-8	dropset
Bent over row	2 x 6-8	dropset
Superset 2	Sets x Reps	
Seated dumbbell overhead press	2 x 8-10	dropset
Incline dumbbell bench press	2 x 8-10	dropset
Superset 3	Sets x Reps	
straight bar tricep pulldown	2 x 8-10	dropset
Bicep curls	2 x 10-12	dropset
Superset 4	Sets x Reps	
close grip pull ups	3 x failure	

Lower body day

Superset 1	Sets x Reps
Squats	2 x 6-8
Leg extension	2 x 15-20
Superset 2	Sets x Reps
Glute bridges	2 x 8-10
Dumbbell lunges	2x 10-12
Superset 3	Sets x Reps
lying/seated Hamstring curls	2 x 10-12
Calf raises	2x 12-15

week schedule

Day	Workout
Monday	Lower Body Workout
Tuesday	walking 45-60mins
Wednesday	60-75% max heart rate cardio of choice for 25 mins
Thursday	Upper Body Workout
Friday	walking 45-60mins
Saturday	60-75% max heart rate cardio of choice for 25 mins
Sunday	20 minute walk

Legs

Superset 1	Sets x Reps	
Leg extension	2 x 6-8	dropset
bodyweight lunges	2 x 6-8	
Superset 2	Sets x Reps	
squats	2 x 8-10	dropset
calf raises	2 x 8-10	dropset
Superset 3	Sets x Reps	
decline crunches	3 x failure	dropset

Back and Biceps

Superset 1	Sets x Reps	
Pull ups	3x failure	
straight bar pullover	2 x 20	dropset
Superset 2	Sets x Reps	
cable rows	2 x 8-10	dropset
lat pull down	2 x 10-15	dropset
Superset 3	Sets x Reps	
Barbell curls	2 x 8-10	dropset
concentration curls	2 x 10-12	dropset

Chest, Shoulders, Triceps

Superset 1	Sets x Reps	
Incline dumbell press	2 x 6-8	dropset
Incline chest fly	2 x 6-8	dropset
Superset 2	Sets x Reps	
cable fly	2 x 8-10	dropset
Lateral raises	2 x 8-10	dropset
Superset 3	Sets x Reps	
Dumbell Overhead press	2 x 8-10	dropset
straight bar tricep pulldown	2 x 10-12	dropset
Superset 4	Sets x Reps	
DIPS	3 x failure	

17

Chest and Back

Superset 1	Sets x Reps	
Flat dumbell press	2 x 10-12	dropset
Supported dumbell row	2 x 10-12	dropset
Superset 2	Sets x Reps	
Incline dumbell flys	2 x 15-20	dropset
underhand pulldowns	2 x 8-10	dropset
Superset 3	Sets x Reps	
Incline Bench press	2 x 8-10	dropset
Cable pullover	2 x 10-12	dropset
Superset 4	Sets x Reps	
push ups	3 x failure	dropset
Pull ups	3 x failure	

Legs and Shoulders

Superset 1	Sets x Reps	
Back squats	2 x 10-12	dropset
Leg extensions	2 x 10-12	dropset
Superset 2	Sets x Reps	
Lying hamstring curls	2 x 15-20	dropset
Calf raises	2 x 8-10	dropset
Superset 3	Sets x Reps	
Dumbell overhead press	2 x 8-10	dropset
Lateral raise	2 x 10-12	dropset
Superset 4	Sets x Reps	
Cable rear delt flq	3 x 25	
EZ bar Upright rows	3 x 25	

Chest and Back

Superset 1	Sets x Reps	
Incline Bench press	2 x 10-12	dropset
underhand pulldowns	2 x 10-12	dropset
Superset 2	Sets x Reps	
Incline dumbell flys	2 x 15-20	dropset
Supported Dumbell rows	2 x 8-10	dropset
Superset 3	Sets x Reps	
Flat dumbell press	2 x 8-10	dropset
Cable pullover	2 x 10-12	dropset
Superset 4	Sets x Reps	
push ups	3 x failure	
Pull ups	3 x failure	

Biceps and Triceps

Superset 1	Sets x Reps	
Straight Bar Pulldown	2 x 10-12	dropset
Dips	2 x failure	
Superset 2	Sets x Reps	
Barbell curls	2 x 15-20	dropset
Concentration curls	2 x 8-10	dropset
Superset 3	Sets x Reps	
supinated chin ups	2 x failure	
Overhead dumbell extension	2 x 10-12	dropset
Superset 4	Sets x Reps	
Decline sit ups	3 x failure	

Chest

Exercise 1	Sets x Reps	
Incline Bench press	2 x 10-12	dropset
Superset 1	Sets x Reps	
Incline chest fly	2 x 15-20	dropset
Flat dumbell press	2 x 8-10	dropset
Exercise 4	Sets x Reps	
dips	3 x failure	

Back

Exercise 1	Sets x Reps	
Close grip Pullups	3 x 10-12	dropset
Superset 1	Sets x Reps	
Lat pulldowns	2 x 15-20	dropset
Cable Pullovers	2 x 20-25	dropset
Superset 3	Sets x Reps	
Bent over row or cable row	2 x 8-10	dropset

legs

Exercise 1	Sets x Reps	
Back squats	2 x 10-12	dropset
Superset 1	Sets x Reps	
Leg extensions	2 x 15-20	dropset
hamstring curls	2 x 8-10	dropset
Exercise 4	Sets x Reps	
Single leg calf raise	3 x failure	

Shoulders

Exercise 1	Sets x Reps	
Dumbell OHP	2 x 10-12	dropset
Superset 1	Sets x Reps	
Lateral raises	2 x 15-20	dropset
cable rear delt fly	2 x 8-10	dropset
Exercise 4	Sets x Reps	
Rope face pull	2 x 12-15	dropset

Arms

Superset 1	Sets x Reps	
Supinated chin ups	3X Failure	
Dips	3X Failure	
Superset 2	Sets x Reps	
Straight arm pulldown	2 x 10-15	dropset
Overhead extension	2 x 8-10	dropset
Superset 3	Sets x Reps	
Barbell Curl	3 x failure	dropset
Concentration curl		dropset

3 BEYOND THE GLASS

The decision to exclusively consume water for the next 66 days is a conscious choice, a reset of your relationship with beverages. This isn't about limiting yourself; it's about freeing yourself—from the amount of sugary indulgences, from the confusion of numerous beverage choices, and from the distractions that can shift you away from the simplicity of genuine hydration. Regard it as a pledge to purity, a dedication to revitalising your body and mind with the fundamental gift of nature.

"So, Josh, how do we determine the right amount of water to drink?" It's quite simple. For every 30 minutes of activity, add 12 ounces of water to your total daily hydration. The baseline is half your weight, and that's the number of ounces of water you should consume each day. For instance, if you weigh 180 pounds, your daily water intake would be 90 ounces, and you add extra the 12 ounces for each 30-minute session. If we really think using common sense, life is impossible without water. Every living organism on Earth requires water for survival. Maintaining proper hydration is a continuous necessity as water plays a crucial role in sustaining life. It has the remarkable ability to alleviate various common issues and body ailments, such as headaches, fatigue, joint pain, and more. While we can endure weeks without food, our survival is limited to just a few days without water. Remarkably, our bodies are composed of approximately 60% water, with the brain and bloodstream holding the highest percentage. Water serves as the fundamental fuel for our bodies, enabling our survival. By prioritising daily hydration, you not only enhance your well-being but also experience increased energy levels.

The primary sources of our water intake include the food we consume and various beverages. While our bodies have the capability to extract water from the food we eat, this process is more intricate compared to simply drinking water. It's essential to note that certain beverages, such as soft drinks and alcohol, lead to significant water loss in the body. Additionally, diuretic drinks like coffee and tea contribute to the depletion of essential nutrients, exacerbating the challenge of maintaining optimal hydration levels.

I've stated the vital role water plays in sustaining life, and now I'll delve into how it actively contributes keeping us alive. Water transports essential nutrients within the body. This role encompasses facilitating proper digestion, aiding in nutrient absorption, and supporting various chemical reactions. Carbohydrates and proteins, integral components of our dietary intake, undergo metabolism and are transported into the bloodstream through the medium of water. Moreover, water assumes a vital role in overall bodily functions, and its absence is the primary trigger for daytime fatigue. Even a minimal 2% decrease in the body's water levels can hinder performance in basic tasks and impede focus while engaging in activities such as reading.

Water serves as a crucial regulator for our body's cooling system. When your body temperature rises, triggering the need to cool down, it relies on the process of sweating. However, for this mechanism to function efficiently, a reserve of water is essential. To illustrate, if you consume 12 ounces of water, your body can absorb 8 ounces of it within a mere 15-minute timeframe. This rapid absorption ensures that your body has the necessary hydration to facilitate the cooling process through sweating when required.

Funny enough, by consistently increasing your water intake, you actively allow the process of removing toxins from your body. The digestive tract, a crucial organ for nutrient absorption and waste elimination, particularly thrives on the benefits of a well-hydrated system. Adequate water intake not only aids in the natural suppression of appetite but also facilitates the body's efficient metabolism off stored fat, fostering a more dynamic and responsive metabolic function. A relatable issue faced by many, is the common confusion between thirst and hunger. To address this often-misunderstood signal, adopting the practice of drinking a full glass of water right 30-45 minutes before a meal proves to be a straightforward yet powerful strategy. Beyond the immediate hydration it provides, this ritual aids in controlling portion sizes, preventing overeating during meals. In this way, incorporating the habit of pre-meal hydration not only satisfies thirst but also becomes a practical tool for mindful and moderated eating, contributing to your overall well-being.

Dehydration doesn't only happen on in hot climates or intense workout sessions; it can creep in stealthily, regardless of the season. Contrary to common misconceptions, the winter season, characterised by cold and dry air, poses a significant risk of dehydration. The chilly air can be deceiving, as the dryness it brings can expedite the body's loss of moisture, potentially leading to dehydration even faster than the sweltering heat of summer. In such conditions, the body's natural mechanisms to regulate temperature, including sweating, may be less noticeable, making it easier to overlook the need for adequate hydration.

Contrary to common perception, dehydration goes beyond its readily noticeable physical symptoms. It can influence other aspects of our well-being, such as appetite and energy levels. When dehydrated, individuals may experience increased feelings of fatigue, coupled with a tendency to consume more food. A simple yet effective gauge of your hydration status is to observe the colour of your urine. Dark yellow urine can be indicative of dehydration, while clear urine suggests adequate hydration. Therefore, it's crucial to stay attuned to your body's signals and consistently prioritise hydration, regardless of the external climate or season.

Now that we have established the importance of hydration, we now have to cover the importance in the quality of what we are drinking. The key here is to steer clear of tap water. Certain contaminants in tap water can pose health risks, and it's crucial to be aware of these potential hazards. Arsenic, a natural metalloid present in groundwater, can enter residential tap water through agricultural or industrial pollution or private wells. Arsenic poisoning, also known as arsenicosis, can lead to various health issues, including partial paralysis, numbness in hands and feet, vomiting, nausea, stomach pain and diarrhoea.

Fluoride, a mineral found in teeth, bones, air, rocks, plants, soil, and water, which can lead to health issues if consumed in excess from tap water. Fluorosis, characterised by mild discolouration of the teeth due to excessive fluoride intake, is one such problem. Additionally, heavy metals like mercury, lead, copper, chromium, cadmium, and aluminum, which may contaminate tap water, can pose long-term health risks. For instance, excessive aluminum intake has been associated with brain deformities and neurological disorders. Inorganic compounds like nitrates are frequently found in processed meats like bacon and ham, where they serve as preservatives. Additionally, these compounds occur naturally in tap water as they are present in the air, soil, and water. While nitrates are common in various environments, their potential health effects, particularly in excessive amounts, have raised concerns.

One of the most controversial health impacts associated with the overconsumption of nitrates is methemoglobinemia, a blood disorder characterised by an abnormal increase in methemoglobin levels. Methemoglobinemia occurs when the body produces an excess of methemoglobin, which starts to replace the normal haemoglobin count. This replacement can lead to insufficient oxygen supply to the cells. In my role of assisting individuals in transforming their lives by optimising performance and energy levels through training and nutrition, I consider mineral or alkaline water to be the most beneficial.

4 HUMAN UPGRADE

A daring exploration of self-optimisation, pushing the boundaries of what it means to enhance our biology and elevate our human capability. The concept of '66 Days' is not arbitrary; it is rooted in the idea that habits are formed over a consistent period, and during these 66 days, we will delve into a series of biohacks designed to reshape our daily rituals and unlock the extraordinary potential within. The rule for this method is just by choosing a minimum of 1 biohack depending on your availability.

Biohacking, at its core, is the science of optimising one's biological systems for improved performance, resilience, and well-being. Our primary goal is to push through these methods without making excuses, as they not only work very well, but are also wallet-friendly and easily adaptable to your daily routine. No need for elaborate justifications or intricate planning; these strategies are made to seamlessly fit into your everyday life. So, discard any excuses, embrace the simplicity, and uncover the potential for positive change that lies within these accessible and straightforward biohacks. It's time to prioritise your well-being without straining your budget or schedule!

I find that the key lies in consistency and commitment rather than overwhelming yourself with an exhaustive list of things to do. By incorporating even, a single biohack into your routine, you open the door to transformation. Whether it's a tweak to your morning routine or a mindful practice before bed, the cumulative effect over 66 days can lead to a remarkable shift in your well-being. This journey is a testament to the power of small, intentional changes, illustrating that even the seemingly minor adjustments can pave the way for a more optimised and vibrant life.

Cold water therapy, ranging from cold showers to cryo chambers, has been a longstanding practice among athletes aiming to expedite post-training recovery. Recently, this approach has gained unprecedented popularity, with certain experts touting it as the ultimate biohack. Experts now state that cold water therapy may activate virus-fighting cells, trigger cold thermogenesis, and potentially extend one's lifespan. Given the widespread availability of cold water, it's emerging as a compelling addition to a health-conscious lifestyle.

Certain studies indicate that exposure to cold water prompts cold thermogenesis, activating brown fat cells. These cells generate heat in colder environments, consequently elevating your overall metabolic rate. Intriguing research has delved into the connection between long-distance cold water swimmers and the stimulation of brown fat cells. Immersing oneself in cold water stimulates leukocytes, the white blood cells crucial for combating infections and viruses. Cold exposure also induces contraction in the lymphatic system, facilitating the flow of fluid through the lymph nodes.

Exposure to cold water or cryotherapy involves a temporary constriction of blood vessels, resulting in a reduction of blood flow to the muscles. This momentary constriction is part of the body's response to the cold stimulus. The reduction in blood flow serves as a protective mechanism to conserve heat and maintain core body temperature. While this vasoconstriction is a short-term effect, it can contribute to long-term improvements in circulation.

The Protocol

A. Start the routine with a regular shower
B. When finished, switch to the coldest setting
C. The goal is to reach 3-5 minutes. If you can't reach that then work your way up each day.
D. Breathe in through your nose and out through your mouth.
E. Close your eyes to relax your mind and body.

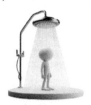

The Sleeping Protocol was simply made to create a natural sense

sense of relaxation. By minimising stressors and creating a tranquil atmosphere, you pave the way for a more serene bedtime routine. When settling into your bed, pay attention to the environmental conditions of your bedroom. Ensure the room is dark and cool, aiming for an ideal temperature between 16°C and 20°C. Creating a comfortable and conducive sleep environment supports the body's natural sleep mechanisms, encouraging a more comfortable night's sleep.

Improve the quality of your sleep by adopting a mindful approach in the hours leading up to bedtime. Refrain from consuming any food within three hours of bedtime, allowing your digestive system to settle and promoting a more restful sleep experience. Additionally, be conscious of the impact of light on your sleep-wake cycle. Minimise exposure to stimulating light impulses, especially from screens, during the last two hours before sleep. Consider using blue-light-blocking glasses to mitigate the disruptive effects of screen time on melatonin production, contributing to a smoother transition into sleep. Additionally, consider waking up to natural light by opening a curtain.

Engage in activities that promote calmness, such as reading a book or practicing gentle stretching exercises. By minimising stressors that you have encountered for the week or day, it will create a calming atmosphere.

The Protocol

A. Stop eating 3 hours before bed
B. Switch off the screens 2-3 hours before bed
C. Keep your room cool at 16-20°C.

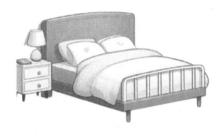

Grounding is establishing contact with the negatively charged Earth h to offer a range of health benefits, primarily through the reduction of oxidative stress. Oxidative stress, an issue characterised by an imbalance between free radicals and the body's ability to neutralise them. This has been linked to the accelerated aging process. Engaging in the simple yet profound act of direct contact with the Earth facilitates an ion exchange, enabling electrons to flow. This remarkable exchange of ions can be effortlessly achieved by activities such as walking barefoot in a forest or immersing yourself in a natural body of water. These interactions with the Earth's surface, sometimes referred to as "earthing" or "grounding," provide a direct pathway for the transfer of electrons from the Earth to the body.

Whether it's the soft grass beneath your feet or the soothing embrace of a natural body of water, the benefits of direct contact with the Earth extend beyond the physical sensations. This connection promotes a harmonious exchange of energy, allowing individuals to tap into the Earth's natural reservoir of electrons. By incorporating these simple practices into daily life, individuals can potentially harness the power of nature to counteract oxidative stress, fostering a sense of balance and well-being.

The potential positive influence on sleep quality, particularly when incorporated into doing this in the evening. The use of the ground or similar items designed to facilitate a direct connection with the Earth's surface holds promise in contributing to an enhancement of the body's circadian rhythm, which, in turn, may lead to a more restful and rejuvenating sleep experience.

The circadian rhythm, often referred to as the body's internal clock, plays a pivotal role in regulating various physiological processes, including sleep-wake cycles. Establishing a connection with the Earth during sleep through grounding could potentially align the body with natural environmental cues. This alignment may, in turn, optimise the circadian rhythm, potentially leading to improved sleep quality.

The Protocol

A. In the evening expose barefoot for 20-30 minutes in a natural environment.

Natural light sets the stage for your wellness routine. Incorporate moments of sun exposure during the morning, noon, and evening, allowing your skin to soak in the revitalising rays for 10 to 15 minutes in the afternoon. Optimise this by ensuring as much skin as possible is exposed, especially when the sun is positioned higher than 42° in the sky. If your shadow is shorter, it indicates that the sun is positioned in a way that facilitates the production of vitamin D in your skin. This is a simple observational method to ensure that you are getting beneficial sun exposure for vitamin D synthesis.

Elevating vitamin D levels through exposure to sunlight is an amazing approach with numerous health benefits. Vitamin D, a vital nutrient, contributes to the promotion of bone health by facilitating the absorption of calcium. This essential function not only fortifies bone density but also contributes to overall skeletal well-being. Beyond its role in bone health, vitamin D emerges as a supporter of immune function, effectively lowering the risk of infections.

Maintaining adequate vitamin D levels has been linked to a decreased likelihood of developing chronic diseases, particularly cardiovascular conditions. The far-reaching impact of vitamin D on the cardiovascular system underscores its significance in supporting heart health. By embracing sunlight as a natural source of this essential vitamin, individuals may fortify their overall health. Although we cover blue light very soon, often emitted by electronic devices, can interfere with the body's production of melatonin, a hormone that regulates sleep. Minimising exposure to blue light in the evening can contribute to better sleep quality, improved circadian rhythm, and overall well-being.

The Protocol

B. Aim for exposure to natural sunlight during morning, noon, and evening for 10-15 mins.
Aim for exposure to natural sunlight during morning, noon, and evening for 10-15 mins.

The Wim Hof Method is a breathing mechanism designed by a Dutch motivational speaker, called Wim Hof. He is known for his ability to endure low temperatures, therefore he has become a notable figure for his unique breathing method. This distinctive approach is recognised for its ability to induce respiratory acidosis, a physiological condition characterised by an excess of carbon dioxide in the blood. Intriguingly, this method operates in stark contrast to the conventional diving response, a natural reaction that typically involves the constriction of blood vessels, elevated blood pressure, and a slower heart rate.

In his unconventional practice, the deliberate induction of respiratory acidosis deviates from the norm, steering the physiological response towards a different outcome. Rather than the expected cardiovascular adjustments associated with the diving response, this method promotes the release of concentrated red blood cells into the bloodstream. Theoretically, this distinctive process holds the potential to enhance athletic performance by ensuring a heightened presence of oxygen-carrying red blood cells.

The Protocol

C. Find a comfortable position.
D. Breathe in deeply through the nose or mouth and through the belly to the chest. Then let the breath go unforced.
E. Exhale through the mouth, then immediately breathe in again.
F. Take 30-40 breaths in short bursts.
G. Take one final, deep inhalation then let the air out and stop inhaling. Hold the breath until you feel the urge to breathe again.
H. Inhale very deeply to full capacity and hold for 15 seconds, then let it go. This completes the first round.
I. Repeat the process between 2-6 times
J. If you have the time after, it is recommended that you meditate and relax.

*Don't do this if you have suffered from a traumatic brain injury recently or ever before. Please first consult with your specialist or doctor.

Forest Bathing, an idea that might seem a bit unusual, involves taking a bath surrounded by nature. Instead, opt for a different kind of immersion—immerse yourself in the beauty of the woods with a stroll through the trees for an hour or two each week. It's especially beneficial to go on this forest walk solo, ensuring an undistracted connection with nature—make it a point to leave your mobile and other gadgets behind. This practice holds advantages for everyone, offering a mental reset and a break from the constant digital buzz.

If feel very brave, try going barefoot for a few steps, or embrace the occasional tree hug for that grounding experience and ion exchange we discussed earlier. These simple acts can enhance your connection with the Earth and contribute to a sense of serenity. However, if you're seeking to elevate your forest immersion, consider venturing out during misty or rainy weather. During these conditions, the air is enriched with terpenes, intensifying the experience and amplifying the therapeutic benefits of your walk. When humans are exposed to phytoncides, typically by spending time in wooded areas or forests, these compounds can have various positive effects on the body. One notable impact is on stress reduction.
Phytoncides have been found to influence the activity of the parasympathetic nervous system, often referred to as the "rest and digest" system. This leads to a decrease in sympathetic nervous system activity, which may lead to reduced stress levels.

The Protocol

K. 20-40 minutes walk in the forest each day.
L. Leave you phone in the car or switch it off completely in a bag
Relax and enjoy your walk.

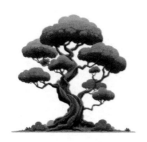

Intermittent fasting, represents a conscious and strategic eating pattern, characterised by the deliberate alternation between periods of eating and fasting. This involves the establishment of specific timeframes dedicated to consuming all daily calories, known as the eating window, and periods of intentional abstention from calorie intake, referred to as the fasting window.

Intermittent fasting has demonstrated its potential to mitigate risks associated with prevalent health concerns. Studies indicate a correlation between intermittent fasting and a decreased likelihood of developing conditions such as diabetes, heart disease, and Alzheimer's. This suggests that embracing this intentional eating pattern could potentially serve as a proactive measure in safeguarding long-term health.

One prominent mechanism is the activation of autophagy, a cellular recycling process stimulated during fasting. Autophagy plays a pivotal role in clearing out damaged cells and promoting the regeneration of new, healthy ones, effectively eliminating inflammatory byproducts. Simultaneously, intermittent fasting has been associated with an elevation in the levels of norepinephrine, a neurotransmitter and hormone. Norepinephrine plays a role in mobilising energy stores, including the breakdown of fats for fuel. This shift towards utilising stored fats helps spare amino acids, the building blocks of proteins, which would otherwise be used for energy.

I adhere to the 16/8 strategy, which is the most commonly practiced form of intermittent fasting. In this routine, I will observe a 16-hour fasting period from 6 p.m. to 10 a.m., abstaining from calorie consumption. During the subsequent 8-hour eating window, typically from 10 a.m. to 6 p.m. During the time of eating, I will consume 3-4 full meals.

The Protocol

M. Establish your period for consuming all daily calories
N. Pay attention to how your body responds.
O. If you have a headache, it might be because your sodium levels are low, therefore drink a 12 ounce glass of water with a pinch of salt or a zero calorie electrolyte powder.

The Sauna Protocol is a heat therapy that has gained attention for its potential health benefits. In the realm of wellness practices, saunas, traditional spaces for heat therapy, have been embraced for centuries across various cultures. Characterised by high temperatures and low humidity, saunas create an environment that induces sweating and provides a range of advantages for both physical and mental well-being. The sustained popularity of saunas reflects the acknowledgment of the beneficial effects that heat therapy can exert on both the body and mind.

Post-workout, it becomes imperative to prioritise muscle relaxation and stretching, essential elements that contribute to the wholesome recovery of engaged muscles. The stress and breakdown of muscle fibres during exercise set the stage for subsequent healing, promoting muscle growth and heightened strength. To optimise this recovery phase, fostering a warm environment is key, as it facilitates muscle relaxation and aids in the overall post-workout recovery process.

Engaging in a post-exercise routine that includes spending a brief yet beneficial 20 minutes in a steam sauna offers an effective strategy. This practice not only induces a sense of relaxation but also serves as a natural mechanism to encourage sweating. Sweating, in turn, becomes a vital means of eliminating toxins accumulated in the body during the day. This deliberate sweating process, facilitated by the heat of the sauna, proves especially advantageous for detoxifying after occasions of indulgence, such as holidays or periods of excess.

The Protocol

P. Shower first, then dry off
Q. Hop into the sauna for 10-15 minutes
R. Take a cold shower or plunge for 3 minutes
S. Take a break to cool off for 30-45 minutes(only if doing another session)

If you are doing this less than 3 times per week, repeat this process twice. If you are doing it, everyday, then it is suggested that you do it once. chapter six text here.

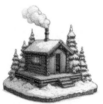

5 THE POWER HOUR

Dedicating an intentional hour each day over the course of the 66 days to learning a new skill can significantly impact both mental and physical well-being. In terms of mental health, this consistent practice stimulates the brain, fostering the creation of new neural connections. As a result, cognitive functions such as memory, problem-solving, and critical thinking are enhanced. The sense of accomplishment derived from visible progress over the dedicated period contributes to increased confidence and an overall positive mental state.

The process of creating new neural connections, known as neuroplasticity, involves the brain's ability to adapt and reorganise itself in response to learning and experience. When you dedicate time each day to learning a new skill, particularly over an extended period like 66 days, this process becomes more pronounced.

Neuroplasticity occurs through a series of complex cellular and molecular changes in the brain. When you engage in learning, whether it's acquiring a new skill or learning something new, neurons in the brain form connections, or with one another. This synaptic connectivity strengthens as you repeatedly practice and reinforce what you're learning.

Over the 66-day period, the consistent and focused nature of your learning sessions reinforces these neural connections. This results in a tangible improvement in cognitive functions associated with the newly acquired skill. Essentially, the brain adapts its neural network to accommodate the demands of the learning process, showcasing the plasticity that allows it to continuously evolve and adapt throughout life.

Creating a plan is the foundational step toward a successful Power Hour, turning what might initially seem like a daunting task into a structured and achievable endeavour. The importance of planning cannot be overstated, as it forms the backbone of your skill acquisition journey. The first critical aspect in this process is the establishment of clear goals. These goals act as the compass, providing a sense of direction and purpose to your learning efforts. Whether you're aiming to learn a new programming language, master a musical instrument, or enhance your language proficiency, setting specific, measurable, achievable, relevant, and time-bound (SMART) goals is key. They not only define your destination but also serve as milestones to gauge your progress.

Once the goals are in place, the next vital component of your plan is to craft a roadmap. This plan outlines the necessary steps to achieve your goals. It acts as a blueprint for your journey, breaking down the goals into manageable tasks and milestones. The roadmap not only ensures a logical progression but also aids in effective time management and resource allocation. With a well-defined roadmap, you gain clarity on the path ahead, making your Power Hour more purposeful and conducive to consistent skill development.

Breaking down your learning into manageable tasks is the third pillar of an effective plan. This involves dissecting your overarching goals into smaller, achievable segments that can be tackled during each Power Hour session. This approach not only minimises the overwhelming nature of skill acquisition but also allows for a more sustainable and rewarding learning experience. Small victories in each session contribute to a sense of accomplishment, fostering motivation and commitment to the Power Hour routine. Furthermore, breaking tasks into smaller parts makes it easier to spot specific areas that might need extra attention and improvement.

In a nutshell, when you build a good foundation through planning, you're not just improving your Power Hour—you're building habits of focus and discipline that stick around even outside your dedicated learning time.

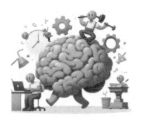

SMART goals serve as a crucial tool in preventing burnout and promoting a sustainable pace of progress. The specific, measurable, achievable, relevant, and time-bound nature of SMART goals inherently encourages a balanced and realistic approach to personal and professional development. Incorporating the SMART criteria into goal-setting practices not only enhances the clarity and achievability of objectives but also promotes an organised approach to personal development.

The "S" in SMART emphasises the importance of precision in goal setting. Rather than vague or general objectives, specific goals clearly define what needs to be accomplished. For instance, instead of setting a goal to "get in shape," a specific goal would be "to jog for 30 minutes five times a week." The specificity of the goal provides a clear target, making it easier to plan and track progress.

The "M" underscores the need for measuring progress. Measurable goals provide a quantifiable way to track progress and determine when the goal has been achieved. Using the previous example, "jogging for 30 minutes five times a week" is measurable because it allows for easy tracking of the frequency and duration of the activity. This element adds a level of accountability and enables everyone to celebrate milestones along the way, which will provide a sense of fulfilment.

The "A" prompts consideration of feasibility. Goals should be challenging but realistic. Setting objectives that are unattainable can lead to frustration and demotivation. An achievable goal takes into account the resources, skills, and time available, ensuring that success is within reach. It will encourage you to stretch your capabilities without setting yourself up for failure or injury.

The "R" emphasises the significance of aligning goals with broader objectives and personal values. A relevant goal is meaningful and contributes to overall growth or desired outcomes. Before committing to a goal, individuals should assess whether it is relevant to their long-term aspirations and whether achieving it will have a positive impact on their lives.

The "T" brings in a time-related element, emphasising the importance of setting deadlines. Without a timeframe, goals may lack urgency and direction. A time-bound goal specifies when the objective should be achieved, creating a sense of urgency and providing a clear endpoint for evaluation. This time constraint also aids in preventing procrastination and encourages consistent effort.

Learning a language in a relatively short span of 66 days may not guarantee fluency, but it can certainly lead to a significant level of knowledge, as by my experience with learning Spanish. In this condensed timeframe, the focus shifts towards practical communication skills, allowing for meaningful conversations and interactions while travelling in Spain. text here. Each day becomes a small section of focused language learning, where the goals are clear, the activities are varied, and the commitment is unwavering. The compact timeline necessitates a strategic approach to the intensity in the Power Hour.

First, I changed my phone's language settings to Spanish, creating an immersive environment where I encountered the language regularly in everyday tasks. This helped in familiarising myself with common phrases and terms encountered in a typical day.

Additionally, I leveraged language-learning apps to streamline my efforts. One key strategy was memorising the 1000 most common words in Spanish. This foundational vocabulary formed the basis for communication and understanding. Apps with interactive features allowed me to practice these words in various contexts, reinforcing their usage in different scenarios.

Consistency was key to my success. Daily practice, whether through dedicated study sessions, listening to podcasts, or watching Spanish content, ensured a steady and gradual improvement. This comprehensive approach, utilising language apps alongside real-world application, contributed to a well-rounded and practical understanding of Spanish within the 66 days.

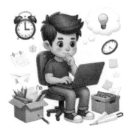

Promoting mental agility,
over the course of 66 days unveils a bunch of cognitive benefits that extend far beyond the acquisition of knowledge. By dedicating a hour each day to intentional learning, you can unlock your intellectual potential. This commitment becomes a catalyst for the enhancement of mental agility, as the brain is continually engaged and challenged, forging new neural pathways and reinforcing existing ones.

As the days progress, the synergy between dedication and cognitive growth becomes increasingly evident, fostering a profound transformation in the your mindset. In the daily grind of learning , creativity gets a good breeding ground to grow. The brain, stuck in the same old routine before, now loves diving into fresh ideas and thinking up new stuff. This newfound creativity isn't just because of sticking to learning every day but also turns out to be a pretty handy tool in work, personal endeavours, and when you're dealing with tricky problems.

 On top of that, getting better at solving problems just happens naturally when you're putting your brain through its paces every day. Dealing with new concepts and tackling brain teasers makes you tougher and more adaptable. Day after day, problem-solving becomes part of how your brain works, giving you the skills to handle tricky situations with confidence and skill. So, that 66-day stretch turns out to be a melting pot not just for loading up on info but also for getting smarter about how to use your brain in real-life situations.

As you embrace the daily challenge of expanding your skillset, you will unfold the layers of cognitive potential, cultivating mental agility, nurturing creativity, and honing problem-solving skills that resonate far beyond the confines of the so called "Power Hour". The 66 days become a small scale of your maximum intellectual potential, marking not only a milestone in time but a profound chapter in the ongoing growth of your personal and cognitive development.

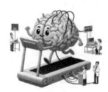

Struggling with ideas on what to learn? Learning isn't just confined to the realm of textbooks and classrooms. Technically you are learning something by reading my books. The world is a playground for acquiring new skills and knowledge, and the possibilities are endless.

Combat sport, beyond physical fitness, instills discipline, focus, and self-confidence, while tennis not only improves physical fitness but also fosters social connections through shared matches and friendly competitions. These diverse pursuits emphasise that education is not confined to classrooms; instead, it thrives in the richness of experiences and the mastery of varied skills. Whether it's shaping wood, perfecting a backhand, or correct your jab technique, the learning journey is an ever-expanding exploration of personal interests, passions, and the boundless possibilities that life has to offer.

In conclusion, the realm of learning is endless, extending far beyond the conventional education systems. The world is offering you an endless opportunity to acquire new skills and knowledge. From the development of discipline through various physical activities to the forging of social connections in shared endeavours, the journey of education is a dynamic exploration of life's diverse aspects. Whether you delve into creative pursuits, refining practical skills, or embracing new passions, the uncharted territory of personal growth unfolds infinitely, unveiling a universe of potential and discovery.

6 SELF REFLECTION

The concept is simple yet profound – each morning, you are encouraged to capture three photographs: one of your face, one of your torso, and one of your back. This seemingly straightforward routine, when woven into the fabric of daily life, unfolds as a powerful tool for introspection and self-awareness. The reason for this is to show as visual documentation accumulates, you embark on a visual timeline of growth and progress. The face becomes a mirror of changing emotions, the torso a canvas illustrating physical well-being, and the back a testament to resilience and overcoming challenges.

Self-reflection isn't about just taking photos, it involves delving deeper into one's own thoughts and experiences. The next 66 days is your chance to use self-reflection as your trusty guide. As you have been reading these pages, let your thoughts wander a bit. Perhaps you can ask yourself. What core values truly drive my decisions and actions, and am I aligning my daily choices with these values? How am I nurturing my personal growth, and what steps can I take today to challenge myself and evolve further? Self-reflection isn't just a checklist of what you're good or bad at. It's about catching those subtle things that make you, well, you. Like, what makes you tick? What weird habits do you have? Embrace the messy parts, the contradictions that make you a unique mix.

 I want YOU to get to the core of why you do what you do, what scares you, and what makes you bounce back after a setback. This self-reflection gig is like having a backstage pass to your own show – the good, the bad, and maybe the slightly weird.

As you encounter setbacks, take a moment to pause and reflect. This pause is a crucial step in understanding the issues of the situation. What went wrong? What lessons can be learned? It is through this reflective process that setbacks become mirrors, offering insights into yourself and the journey ahead.

Resilience is the cornerstone of turning setbacks into stepping stones. Rather than viewing failure as an endpoint, change the mindset that perceives it as feedback, a stepping stone toward improvement. Embrace the wisdom of Vince Lombardi, "It's not whether you get knocked down, it's whether you get up." Setbacks demand adaptability. Use them as an advantage to reassess your strategies and make necessary adjustments. Recognise that progress is often incremental, and setbacks are integral to the journey. Celebrate not just the destination but the small victories along the way. Remember, as Winston Churchill aptly put it, "Success is stumbling from failure to failure with no loss of enthusiasm."

Embarking on the journey of self-reflection requires a courageous spirit, a readiness to confront one's innermost thoughts and emotions with vulnerability. In the topic of self-discovery, acknowledging vulnerability as a potent force is paramount. Rather than shying away from it, recognise it as the cornerstone of authenticity. By navigating the challenges presented in the book with an open heart and mind, you allow vulnerability to guide you toward a deeper understanding of yourself. In this process, you not only connect with the narrative but also forge a more intimate relationship with your own journey of growth. It's crucial to realise the misconception that vulnerability equates to fragility. On the contrary, it is a wellspring of strength that empowers you to face the complexities of your emotions and experiences. As you courageously change your life in 66 days, remember that each moment of vulnerability is a stepping stone towards genuine authenticity and a richer comprehension of your own narrative.

A habit of self-reflection is much like constructing a solid foundation for a building—one that supports the structure of personal growth and heightened self-awareness. This analogy emphasises the importance of a stable base upon your self-development can rise and stand resilient against the challenges of everyday life. In the same way that a well-built foundation is crucial for the stability and longevity of a house, regular self-reflection forms the bedrock of your personal evolution.

Consider the morning fasted cardio routine as the groundbreaking phase of your self-reflection construction project. It is here that you lay the initial bricks, setting the tone for the day. Morning reflections act as the cornerstone, providing stability and direction as you navigate the challenges and opportunities that arise. This intentional beginning fosters a sense of purpose, much like the commencement of construction marks the initiation of a building's rise.

The evening then becomes the phase of final touches—a time for thorough inspection and adjustment. Your evening reflections are akin to the finishing details that complete a building, refining its aesthetics and functionality. Delving into the events of the day, expressing gratitude, and identifying areas for improvement contribute to the overall solidity and resilience of your self-reflective foundation.

Aligning your actions with your values during this challenge adds a layer to your experience. It transforms the act of reading into a mindful journey where each page turned becomes a conscious step towards personal improvement.

Moreover, examining the alignment between your actions and values in the context of this challenge extends beyond the aspect of reading this last chapter. It prompts you to evaluate the intentionality behind your choices, fostering self-awareness and a deeper understanding of what truly matters to you. This awareness can serve as an advantage to other factors of your life, influencing decisions beyond the scope of The 66 Change.

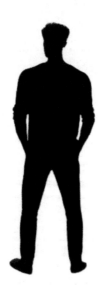

7 CONCLUSION

The essence of this narrative lies in the empowerment it provides—equipping you with knowledge and tools to orchestrate a comprehensive transformation. I've delved into strategies that extend beyond adjustments, aiming to fundamentally alter your habits, mindset, and, consequently, your entire life.

This journey is not just about the passage of time; it is about intentional growth and a transformative change. Whether you approach it with unwavering determination or occasional hesitations, you've been an active participant in sculpting a better, healthier version of yourself.

Thank you for being part of this transformative change. Your commitment to "The 66 Change" is not just a chapter in a book—it's a testament to your dedication to a healthier, more empowered, and revitalised version of yourself. Until we meet again on the next book unravelling the secrets to this health matrix, may your path be illuminated with newfound knowledge, resilience, and the unwavering pursuit of well-being.

Oh, I didn't mention earlier, but once you've finished your 66 days, if you can, shoot me a video sharing how you're feeling post the journey. Best of luck!

Your Journal

MEALPLAN

Date
_____

	BREAKFAST	LUNCH	DINNER	SNACKS
MON				
TUE				
WED				
THU				
FRI				
SAT				
SUN				

Shopping list

_____ _____ _____
_____ _____ _____
_____ _____ _____
_____ _____ _____
_____ _____ _____

PROGRESS PLAN Date _____

Training Date	Exercise	Sets	Reps	Rest time

Goal:	Answer:
Smart goal:	
What do I want to accomplish?	
Why is this goal important?	
Measureable:	
How will I track my progress?	
How will I know when it's done?	
Achievable:	
Is the goal realistic and attainable?	
Do I have the resources and capabilities to achieve it?	
Relevant:	
Does this goal align with my broader objectives?	
Is it the right time to pursue this goal?	
Time-Bound:	
What is the deadline for achieving this goal?	
What are the milestones along the way?	

WORKOUT PLAN

Date _____

Exercise	Sets x Reps	Advanced technique

Exercise	Sets x Reps	Advanced technique

Exercise	Sets x Reps	Advanced technique

Exercise	Sets x Reps	Advanced technique

Exercise	Sets x Reps	Advanced technique

Challenge Description	Initial Reaction	Positive Approach

The 66 Change

Date	How i physically feel

Date	Type of fasted cardio	Duration

Exercise	Personal reord	Date achieved

Date	Water intake

date	Weight	Current feeling
Week 1		
Week 2		
Week 3		
Week 4		
Week 5		
Week 6		
Week 7		
Week 8		
Week 9		
Week 10		
Week 11		

Date	Sleep quality	Mood	Stress level

date	Wake up time time	Bed time	how you feel

Date	Biohack chosen	Duration (minutes)	Thoughts/Feelings
Day 29			
Day 30			
Day 31			
Day 32			
Day 33			
Day 34			
Day 35			
Day 36			
Day 37			
Day 38			
Day 39			
Day 40			
Da 41			
Day 42			

Date	Biohack chosen	Duration (minutes)	Thoughts/Feelings
Day 15			
Day 16			
Day 17			
Day 18			
Day 19			
Day 20			
Day 21			
Day 22			
Day 23			
Day 24			
Day 25			
Day 26			
Day 27			
Day 28			

Date	Biohack chosen	Duration (minutes)	Thoughts/Feelings
Day 1			
Day 2			
Day 3			
Day 4			
Day 5			
Day 6			
Day 7			
Day 8			
Day 9			
Day 10			
Day 11			
Day 12			
Day 13			
Day 14			

Date	Biohack chosen	Duration (minutes)	Thoughts/Feelings
Day 43			
Day 44			
Day 45			
Day 46			
Day 47			
Day 48			
Day 49			
Day 50			
Day 51			
Day 52			
Day 53			
Day 54			
Day 55			
Day 56			

Date	Biohack chosen	Duration (minutes)	Thoughts/Feelings
Day 57			
Day 58			
Day 59			
Day 60			
Day 61			
Day 62			
Day 63			
Day 64			
Day 65			
Day 66			

The Health Matrix

The concept of the health matrix, as I perceive it, is a web of choices and consequences in one's lifestyle that may lead to declining well-being. It's a narrative that unfolds when individuals neglect crucial aspects of self-care, such as exercise and mindful nutrition, resulting in a gradual descent into ill health and, subsequently, a dependence on medication.

Dietary choices play a pivotal role within this sequence of events. Opting for convenience over nutritional value, becoming over exposed to hidden dangers in processed foods, or maintaining a diet devoid of essential nutrients can significantly contribute to the unfolding health narrative.

As this neglect persists, the sequence evolves. The body, deprived of adequate exercise and proper nutrition, becomes more susceptible to chronic conditions. Weight gain, high blood pressure, and elevated triglyceride levels become unwelcome. The not-so-obvious results of those decisions are now showing up as real health problems, making a trip to the doctor necessary.

Enter the reliance on medications—a consequence of navigating this sequence. Prescribed to manage symptoms and mitigate the impact of preventable health issues, medications become a lifeline for those ensnared in the matrix. The irony lies in the fact that the very dependence on medication underscores a missed opportunity for preventative care—a chance to break free from the clutches of this health narrative.

This narrative is not a judgment but a recognition of a common trajectory that many follow. It is a call to awareness and intentional decision-making. Breaking free from this "Health Matrix" involves acknowledging the importance of regular exercise, making informed dietary choices, and prioritising preventative care to foster lasting well-being.

By recognising this interplay and taking proactive steps towards self-care, individuals have the power to reshape their health trajectory, steering away from dependence on medications and embracing a life characterised by vitality and wellness.

Thank you

The 66 Change

The 66 Change

The 66 Change

The 66 Change

Printed in Great Britain
by Amazon

36074644R00046